EVERYTHING

YOU OUGHT TO KNOW ABOUT

FAT LOSS

By

Roger N. Jackson

This book is dedicated to my Husband, Annalisa and Chrysolite.

You have been my greatest inspiration.

And for every individual who desires to transform their body and cultivate a healthy lifestyle.

You're loved.

Table of Contents

INTRODUCTION

"Welcome to "Everything you ought to know about fat loss," the ultimate guide to achieving your weight loss goals and leading a healthier and happier life. In a world where fad diets and weight loss gimmicks are all too common, this book provides a comprehensive, science-based proven approach to sustainable fat loss. Whether you are just starting your weight loss journey or looking to break through a plateau, "Everything you ought to know about fat loss," offers a wealth of information and practical tips to help you succeed.

Throughout this book, you will learn about the various factors that influence weight loss. You will also gain a deeper understanding of how your body processes and stores fat, and how to use this knowledge to your advantage.

But this book is more than just a collection of facts and figures. "Everything you ought to know about fat loss," is designed to be a practical guide that you can use to make real and lasting changes in your life. You will find simple and actionable steps for improving your diet, increasing your physical activity, and managing stress. You will also learn how to overcome common obstacles to fat loss and maintain your progress over the long term.

At its core, "Everything you ought to know about fat loss," is about empowering you to take control of your health and wellbeing. By arming you with the knowledge and tools you need to achieve your weight loss goals, this book will help you to not only look and feel better, but to live a more fulfilling life. So whether you are looking to shed a few pounds or transform your entire body, "Everything you ought to know about fat loss," is the ultimate resource for anyone who is dedicated to achieving their fitness and health goals.

The information in "Everything you ought to know about fat loss," is based on the latest scientific research and has been carefully curated by experts in the fields of nutrition, exercise physiology, and psychology. You can trust that the advice in this book is evidence-based and backed by years of experience helping people achieve their weight loss goals.

In addition to the practical tips and strategies, "Everything you ought to know about fat loss," also provides motivational guidance and mindset coaching to help you overcome the mental and emotional challenges that often accompany weight loss. You will learn how to stay motivated, set realistic goals, and cultivate a positive self-image that will support your efforts to live a healthy and active lifestyle.

Ultimately, "Everything you ought to know about fat loss," is divided into three parts which will help you achieve a happier, healthier, and more fulfilling life. By improving your physical health and well-being, you will also experience improved energy levels, mental clarity, and overall quality of life. With the information and guidance in this book, you can finally take control of your weight and transform your body and your life. So let's get started!

PART ONE: UNDERSTANDING FAT LOSS

CHAPTER ONE

What is Fat Loss?

Fat loss refers to the process of reducing the amount of body fat in a person's body. This can be achieved through a combination of changes in diet, exercise, and other lifestyle factors. When the body is in a state of negative energy balance, meaning that it is burning more calories than it is consuming, it will begin to break down stored fat to use as energy, which reduces body fat.

Fat loss is often pursued for a variety of reasons, including improved health and fitness, improved body composition, and increased confidence and self-esteem. However, it is important to note that fat loss should not be pursued to the point of extreme or unhealthy weight loss, as this can have negative consequences on a person's physical and mental health.

Overall, fat loss is a complex and multifaceted process that requires a combination of lifestyle changes to achieve sustainable results. By implementing healthy habits and adopting a balanced approach to nutrition and exercise, individuals can achieve healthy and sustainable fat loss while improving their overall health and well-being.

It is important to note that fat loss is not always the same as weight loss. While losing weight does involve losing body fat, it can also involve losing water weight, muscle mass, and other components of the body. This is why it is important to focus on fat loss rather than just overall weight loss.

One way to measure fat loss is by tracking body composition. This involves measuring the percentage of body fat compared to other components, such as muscle mass, bone density, and water weight. Tracking body composition can help you to determine whether you are losing fat or other components of the body, and can help you to adjust your diet and exercise plan accordingly.

It is also important to approach fat loss with a realistic mindset. Sustainable fat loss takes time and effort and it is important to be patient and consistent in your efforts. It is also important to set realistic goals and to avoid comparing yourself to others. The body of each person is unique, so what works for one person might not work for another.

Why is Fat Loss Important?

Fat loss is important for a number of reasons, both physical and mental. Here are some of the key reasons why fat loss is important:

Improved overall health: excess body fat is associated with a range of health problems, including heart disease, type 2 diabetes, and certain types of cancer. By losing body fat, you can reduce your risk of these health issues and improve your overall health.

Improved body composition: excess body fat can also affect your body composition, leading to a higher percentage of body fat and a lower percentage of lean muscle mass. By losing body fat and building lean muscle, you can improve your body composition, which can improve your physical performance, strength, and overall appearance.

Increased energy and vitality: losing body fat can also help to increase your energy levels and vitality. Carrying excess body fat can make it harder to move and be active, whereas losing fat can help you to move more easily and feel more energized.

Improved mental health: carrying excess body fat can also affect your mental health, leading to low self-esteem, poor body image, and other mental health issues. Losing body fat and improving your overall health and fitness can boost your self-confidence and improve your mental health.

Improved quality of life: ultimately, fat loss can lead to an improved quality of life. By improving your health and fitness, you can enjoy more activities, have more energy, and feel better overall.

In addition to the benefits mentioned earlier, fat loss can also help with:

Hormone regulation: excess body fat can disrupt hormone levels in the body, which can have negative impacts on a range of bodily functions, such as metabolism, sleep, and mood. Losing body fat can help to regulate hormone levels and improve overall hormonal balance.

Better sleep: losing body fat can help to reduce snoring, sleep apnea, and other sleep-related issues. It can also improve sleep quality, which can lead to better overall health and well-being.

Increased mobility: excess body fat can restrict movement and make it harder to engage in physical activities. Losing body fat can improve mobility and make it easier to move and exercise, which can lead to further improvements in health and fitness.

Lowered inflammation: fat loss can also help to reduce inflammation in the body, which is linked to a range of health problems, including heart disease, type 2 diabetes, and arthritis.

Lowered risk of injury: carrying excess body fat can increase the risk of injury, particularly in the joints and back. By losing body fat and building lean muscle, you can improve your overall physical function and reduce the risk of injury.

Another important aspect of fat loss is that it can help to increase metabolic rate. Metabolic rate refers to the number of calories the body burns each day to maintain its basic functions, such as breathing and circulating blood. When an individual loses body fat, they may also increase their metabolic rate, as muscle tissue burns more calories than fat tissue.

In other words, losing body fat and building muscle can help to increase the body's overall calorie burn, even when the individual is at rest. This means that an individual who has lost body fat may be able to consume more calories each day without gaining weight, which can make it easier to maintain a healthy weight over the long term.

Furthermore, fat loss can help to improve insulin sensitivity, which is important for managing blood sugar levels. When an individual has excess body fat, their body may become resistant to insulin, which can lead to high blood sugar levels and an increased risk of type 2 diabetes. Losing body fat can help to improve insulin sensitivity, which can lead to better blood sugar control and a reduced risk of diabetes.

In summary, fat loss is the process of reducing body fat through a combination of diet, exercise, and lifestyle changes. By focusing on sustainable, healthy habits and adopting a balanced approach, individuals can achieve healthy and sustainable fat loss while improving their overall health and well-being.

CHAPTER TWO

Science of Fat Loss

The science of fat loss is complex and multifaceted, involving a range of biological and physiological factors. Essentially, fat loss occurs when the body burns more calories than it consumes, leading to a calorie deficit. When the body is in a calorie deficit, it must draw on its fat stores to meet its energy needs, which leads to fat loss over time.

There are several factors that can influence the rate of fat loss, including:

Energy balance: as mentioned earlier, fat loss occurs when the body is in a calorie deficit. This means that an individual must consume fewer calories than they burn in order to lose body fat. Factors that can impact energy balance include diet, exercise, and daily activity levels.

Hormonal balance: hormones play a key role in regulating the body's metabolism and fat storage. Hormones such as insulin, cortisol, and leptin can impact the body's ability to burn fat and maintain a healthy weight.

Genetics: genetics can also play a role in fat loss, as some individuals may be predisposed to carrying more body fat or may have a slower metabolism.

Exercise: exercise can help to increase calorie burn and build lean muscle, both of which can aid in fat loss. High-intensity interval training (HIIT) and strength training are particularly effective for fat loss.

Sleep: Sleep plays an important role in regulating hormones that impact metabolism and appetite. Poor sleep quality or quantity can disrupt these hormonal processes and lead to weight gain and fat storage.

Overall, the science of fat loss is complex and multifaceted, and there are many factors that can impact an individual's ability to lose body fat. By adopting a healthy, balanced approach to diet and exercise, individuals can achieve fat loss and improve their overall health and well-being.

At the cellular level, fat loss involves the breakdown and release of stored fat from adipose tissue. The body stores excess calories as fat in adipose tissue, which can be broken down and used for energy when the body is in a calorie deficit. This process is regulated by hormones, such as adrenaline and noradrenaline, which trigger the breakdown of fat cells and the release of stored fatty acids.

Once fatty acids are released into the bloodstream, they can be taken up and burned for energy by cells throughout the body. The mitochondria within cells are responsible for burning fatty acids to produce energy, which can be used to fuel physical activity and basic bodily functions.

However, the body can also burn muscle tissue for energy, which is why it is important to maintain muscle mass during fat loss. Resistance training and high-protein diets can help to preserve muscle mass while promoting fat loss.

Ultimately, fat loss is a complex process that involves a range of biological and physiological factors. By adopting a healthy, balanced approach to diet and exercise, individuals can support their body's natural fat-burning processes and achieve long-term fat loss and weight management.

Another important aspect of the science of fat loss is the concept of metabolic adaptation. When an individual begins to lose weight and body fat, the body may respond by slowing down its metabolic rate, making it more difficult to continue losing weight. This is because the body perceives a calorie deficit as a threat to survival and adapts by conserving energy.

This can be frustrating for individuals who are trying to lose weight, as it can make weight loss more difficult over time.

However, there are strategies that can be used to mitigate metabolic adaptation and support long-term weight loss.

One strategy is to adopt a gradual approach to weight loss, which can help to prevent a large drop in metabolic rate. Additionally, incorporating regular resistance training into a weight loss program can help to preserve muscle mass and boost metabolic rate, making it easier to continue losing weight.

Another strategy is to periodically increase calorie intake, a technique known as "reverse dieting." By gradually increasing calorie intake over time, individuals can help to reset their metabolic rate and prevent the body from adapting to a calorie deficit.

Overall, the science of fat loss is complex and multifaceted, and there are many factors that can impact an individual's ability to lose weight and body fat. By adopting a sustainable, healthy approach to weight loss, individuals can achieve their goals while supporting their long-term health and well-being.

Metabolism and energy

Metabolism and energy balance play a key role in the body's ability to burn fat and maintain a healthy weight. Metabolism refers to the chemical processes that occur within cells to convert food into energy. The body's metabolic rate is the amount of energy (calories) that the body burns at rest to maintain basic bodily functions. A high metabolic rate can help to burn more calories and aid in weight loss, while a low metabolic rate can make it more difficult to lose weight.

Energy balance refers to the relationship between the calories consumed through food and the calories burned through physical activity and basic bodily functions. When an individual is in a calorie deficit (burning more calories than they consume), the body must draw on its fat stores to meet its energy needs, leading to fat loss over time.

Metabolism and energy are closely related concepts. Metabolism refers to the chemical processes that occur within cells to convert food into energy, while energy refers to the ability to do work. The body's metabolism is responsible for converting the food we eat into energy that can be used to power all of our bodily functions, from basic cellular processes to physical activity.

The body's metabolic rate is the amount of energy (calories) that the body burns at rest to maintain basic bodily functions.

The metabolic rate is influenced by a variety of factors, including age, sex, body composition, genetics, and lifestyle factors such as diet and exercise.

When an individual consumes more calories than they burn, the excess calories are stored as fat, leading to weight gain over time. Conversely, when an individual burns more calories than they consume, the body must draw on its fat stores to meet its energy needs, leading to weight loss over time.

One way to increase the body's metabolic rate is to engage in regular physical activity, which can help to build muscle mass and increase the number of calories burned at rest. High-intensity exercise can also help to boost the body's metabolic rate for several hours after exercise, leading to greater overall calorie burn.

Additionally, eating a healthy, balanced diet can help to support the body's metabolic rate and energy levels. Foods that are high in protein, fiber, and complex carbohydrates can help to boost metabolism and maintain stable energy levels throughout the day.

Another important aspect of metabolism and energy is the concept of the basal metabolic rate (BMR). The BMR is the number of calories that the body burns at rest to maintain basic bodily functions such as breathing, circulation, and digestion.

The BMR is influenced by factors such as age, sex, body composition, and genetics.

Building and maintaining muscle mass can help to increase the BMR, as muscle tissue burns more calories at rest than fat tissue. Additionally, eating a balanced diet that includes adequate protein and carbohydrates can help to support the body's energy needs and maintain stable blood sugar levels throughout the day.

The body's metabolism can also be impacted by medical conditions such as hypothyroidism, which can lead to a slower metabolic rate and difficulty losing weight. In these cases, medical intervention may be necessary to support weight loss and overall health.

A healthy metabolism and energy levels can also have a positive impact on mood, cognitive function, and overall quality of life. By adopting healthy lifestyle habits that support the body's natural metabolic and energy processes, individuals can achieve optimal health and wellness.

CHAPTER THREE

Managing Hormones

Managing hormones is an important aspect of fat loss, as imbalances in certain hormones can make it more difficult to lose weight. Here are some strategies for managing hormones and supporting fat loss:

Manage stress: stress can increase levels of the hormone cortisol, which can lead to weight gain and make it more difficult to lose fat. Strategies for managing stress can include meditation or deep breathing exercises.

Get enough sleep: lack of sleep can disrupt hormone levels and make it more difficult to lose weight. Aim for 7-8 hours of sleep per night to support healthy hormone levels and improve overall health.

Eat a balanced diet: eating a balanced diet that includes a variety of nutrients can help support healthy hormone levels. Eat whole, nutrient-dense foods such as fruits, vegetables, lean proteins, and healthy fats.

Exercise regularly: exercise can help support healthy hormone levels and improve fat loss. Both cardio and resistance training can be effective, and it's important to find activities that you enjoy and can stick to long-term.

Stay hydrated: drinking enough water can help support healthy hormone levels and improve overall health. Target to drink at least 8-10 cups of water a day.

Eat enough protein: adequate protein intake is important for supporting healthy hormone levels and maintaining muscle mass during weight loss. Aim for eight to ten cups of water each day.

Limit alcohol intake: excessive alcohol consumption can disrupt hormone levels and make it more difficult to lose weight. Aim to limit alcohol intake to no more than one drink per day for women and two drinks per day for men.

Manage insulin levels: high levels of insulin can make it difficult to lose weight, so it's important to manage insulin levels by eating a balanced diet that includes complex carbohydrates, healthy fats, and protein. Avoid processed foods and sugary drinks that can cause insulin spikes.

Consider intermittent fasting: Intermittent fasting is a dietary strategy that involves alternating periods of fasting with periods of eating. This can help improve insulin sensitivity and support fat loss.

Get enough vitamin D: Vitamin D is an important nutrient that can help support healthy hormone levels. Aim to get enough vitamin D through sun exposure, fortified foods, or supplements.

Hormones and Fat Storage

Hormones also play a key role in regulating the body's metabolism and fat storage. Insulin is a hormone that regulates the uptake of glucose (sugar) from the bloodstream into cells for energy. High levels of insulin can promote fat storage and make it more difficult for the body to burn fat. Cortisol is a hormone that is released in response to stress, and high levels of cortisol can lead to increased fat storage and a slower metabolism. Leptin is a hormone that regulates appetite and metabolism, and low levels of leptin can make it more difficult to lose weight.

In addition to hormones, there are other factors that can impact the body's ability to burn fat and maintain a healthy weight. These include genetics, age, sex, and lifestyle factors such as diet and physical activity.

Overall, the relationship between metabolism, energy balance, hormones, and fat storage is complex and multifaceted.

Hormones play an important role in regulating fat storage in the body. Insulin, a hormone produced by the pancreas, helps to regulate the uptake of glucose (sugar) from the bloodstream into cells for energy. High levels of insulin can promote fat storage and make it more difficult for the body to burn fat. This is because when insulin levels are high, the body is more likely to store excess glucose as fat rather than use it for energy.

Cortisol is another hormone that is involved in the regulation of fat storage. Cortisol is released in response to stress, and high levels of cortisol can lead to increased fat storage and a slower metabolism. This is because cortisol signals the body to store fat in anticipation of a "fight or flight" response, even if the stressor is not physical in nature.

Leptin is a hormone produced by fat cells that helps to regulate appetite and metabolism. Leptin signals the brain to decrease appetite and increase metabolism when fat stores are high, and to increase appetite and decrease metabolism when fat stores are low. However, in some cases, individuals may become resistant to leptin, which can make it more difficult to lose weight and maintain a healthy body weight.

Other hormones that play a role in regulating fat storage include ghrelin, a hormone that increases appetite and promotes fat storage, and adiponectin, a hormone that helps to regulate insulin sensitivity and promote fat burning.

One hormone that has gained a lot of attention in recent years in relation to fat storage is adiponectin. Adiponectin is produced by fat cells and helps to regulate insulin sensitivity and promote fat burning. Low levels of adiponectin have been linked to obesity, insulin resistance, and other metabolic disorders.

Research has suggested that lifestyle factors such as diet and exercise can impact adiponectin levels. For example, diets that are high in sugar and refined carbohydrates can decrease adiponectin levels, while diets that are high in fiber and healthy fats can increase adiponectin levels.

Similarly, engaging in regular physical activity can help to increase adiponectin levels and support healthy metabolism and fat loss. This may be due to the fact that exercise can help to increase muscle mass, which in turn can help to boost the body's metabolic rate and support healthy fat burning.

Other hormones that have been linked to fat storage include estrogen and testosterone. In women, high levels of estrogen can promote fat storage in the hips and thighs, while low levels of testosterone in men can lead to increased fat storage in the abdominal region.

Overall, the relationship between hormones and fat storage is complex and multifaceted, and may be impacted by a variety of factors such as age, sex, genetics, and lifestyle habits. By adopting a healthy, balanced approach to diet and exercise, individuals can support their body's natural hormonal processes and achieve long-term health and wellness.

Hormones and Hunger

Hormones can play a significant role in regulating hunger and appetite. Here are some hormones that can impact hunger:

Ghrelin: ghrelin is often called the "hunger hormone" because it stimulates appetite and can increase food intake. Ghrelin is produced in the stomach and signals the brain to stimulate hunger before meals and decrease after meals.

Leptin: leptin is a hormone produced by fat cells that signals the brain to decrease appetite and increase energy expenditure. It helps regulate long-term energy balance by signaling the brain that enough energy has been stored and reducing the drive to eat.

Insulin: Insulin:insulin is a hormone produced by the pancreas that helps regulate blood sugar levels. High levels of insulin can increase hunger and cravings for high-carbohydrate foods.

Cortisol: cortisol is a stress hormone that can increase appetite and cravings for high-calorie, high-fat foods. Chronically high cortisol levels can disrupt hunger regulation and contribute to weight gain.

By understanding the impact of these hormones on hunger and appetite, it's possible to develop strategies to manage hunger and support weight loss. Some strategies may include:

Eating protein-rich foods: protein is known to be more satiating than other macro nutrients, and can help reduce levels of ghrelin while increasing levels of leptin.

Eat fiber-rich foods: fiber can help reduce hunger and increase feelings of fullness by slowing down digestion and regulating blood sugar levels. Foods rich in fiber include fruits, vegetables, whole grains, and legumes.

Include healthy fats: healthy fats, such as those found in nuts, seeds, avocados, and fatty fish, can help regulate hormones and reduce hunger.

Eat regularly: skipping meals or going long periods without eating can disrupt hormone levels and increase hunger. Aim to eat regular, balanced meals throughout the day to support healthy hormone levels and reduce cravings.

Avoid processed foods: processed foods that are high in sugar, salt, and unhealthy fats can disrupt hormone levels and increase hunger. Instead, focus on whole, nutrient-dense foods to support healthy hormones and reduce hunger.

Remember, the key to managing hormones and hunger is to focus on overall lifestyle habits that support weight loss and improve overall health. By incorporating healthy eating habits, regular exercise, and stress-management techniques, it's possible to achieve long-term weight loss and improve your overall health and well-being. Consulting with a healthcare professional or registered dietitian can also be helpful for developing a personalized plan that meets your individual needs and goals.

Strategies for Hormone Management

Here are some strategies for hormone management that can support healthy weight loss:

Incorporate strength training: resistance training and weight lifting can help increase lean muscle mass and support healthy hormone levels, including testosterone and growth hormone. This can also help increase metabolism and support fat loss.

Avoid crash dieting: crash dieting or severe calorie restriction can disrupt hormone levels and lead to muscle loss and a slower metabolism. Instead, focus on gradual, sustainable weight loss through a balanced diet and regular exercise.

Get enough sleep: lack of sleep can disrupt hormone levels, including cortisol and ghrelin, which can increase hunger and disrupt metabolism. Aim for at least 7-8 hours of sleep per night to support healthy hormone levels and weight loss.

Manage stress: chronic stress can disrupt hormone levels, including cortisol, insulin, and thyroid hormones, which can contribute to weight gain and difficulty losing weight. Incorporating stress-management techniques, such as meditation, yoga, or deep breathing exercises, can help support healthy hormone levels and weight loss.

Eat a balanced diet: a balanced diet that includes a variety of nutrient-dense foods can help support healthy hormone levels and weight loss. Include plenty of fruits, vegetables, whole grains, lean protein, and healthy fats in your diet to support healthy hormone levels and weight loss.

Reduce exposure to toxins: exposure to environmental toxins, such as pesticides, herbicides, and plastics, can disrupt hormone levels and contribute to weight gain. To reduce exposure, choose organic produce, use natural cleaning products, and avoid heating food in plastic containers.

Eat enough protein: protein is important for supporting healthy hormone levels and muscle growth. Include sources of lean protein, such as chicken, fish, beans, and lentils, in your diet to support healthy hormones and weight loss.

Include probiotics: probiotics can help support healthy gut bacteria and improve digestion, which can in turn support healthy hormone levels and weight loss. Include sources of probiotics, such as yogurt, kefir, kimchi, or sauerkraut, in your diet.

Avoid artificial sweeteners: artificial sweeteners, such as aspartame and sucralose, can disrupt hormone levels and contribute to weight gain. Avoid or limit intake of products that contain artificial sweeteners to support healthy hormone levels and weight loss.

Use healthy cooking oils: cooking with healthy oils, such as olive oil, avocado oil, or coconut oil, can support healthy hormone levels and weight loss. Avoid using oils that are high in trans fats, such as vegetable oil or shortening.

CHAPTER FOUR

Role of Exercise and Diet

Exercise and diet play crucial roles in achieving and maintaining weight loss. Here are some of the specific roles that exercise and diet play in the book:

Exercise helps burn calories and increase metabolism: The book explains that regular exercise can help burn calories and increase metabolism, which can aid in weight loss. Exercise can also help build muscle, which can help burn more calories even at rest.

Diet controls calorie intake: By consuming fewer calories than your body burns, you create a calorie deficit that can lead to weight loss. The book also recommends focusing on whole, nutrient-dense foods that are low in calories but high in nutrients.

Exercise and diet together create a larger calorie deficit: you create a larger calorie deficit, which can lead to more significant weight loss. I recommend finding a balance between the two that works for you and your lifestyle.

Exercise and diet can improve overall health: regular exercise and a healthy diet can reduce the risk of chronic diseases such as diabetes, heart disease, and certain types of cancer.

Exercise and diet can improve mood and reduce stress: exercise releases endorphins, which are natural mood boosters, while a healthy diet provides the nutrients needed for optimal brain function.

Exercise and diet can help with sleep: regular exercise can help regulate the sleep-wake cycle, while a healthy diet can provide the nutrients needed for restful sleep.

Exercise and diet can boost energy levels: exercise increases circulation and oxygen flow, while a healthy diet provides the nutrients needed for optimal energy production.

Exercise and diet can improve body composition: this means the ratio of lean muscle mass to body fat. By building muscle and reducing body fat, you can achieve a leaner, more toned physique.

Exercise and diet can help create healthy habits: by making regular exercise and healthy eating a part of your lifestyle, you can maintain weight loss and overall health.

The Impact of Exercise and Diet

The impact of exercise and diet on health and fat loss is significant. Here are some of the ways that exercise and diet can impact your health and weight loss:

Improved cardiovascular health: regular exercise and a healthy diet can improve cardiovascular health by reducing the risk of heart disease, lowering blood pressure and cholesterol levels, and improving blood flow.

Improved metabolic health: exercise and a healthy diet can improve metabolic health by increasing insulin sensitivity, which can help prevent and manage diabetes, and improving liver function, which can aid in fat loss.

Increased weight loss: exercise and a healthy diet create a calorie deficit, which can lead to weight loss. By burning more calories through exercise and consuming fewer calories through a healthy diet, you can achieve significant weight loss.

Increased muscle mass: exercise can help increase muscle mass, which can lead to an increase in metabolism and the ability to burn more calories even at rest.

Reduced body fat: a healthy diet and regular exercise can reduce body fat, which can improve overall health and reduce the risk of chronic diseases such as diabetes and heart disease.

Improved bone density: exercise, especially weight-bearing exercise, can improve bone density, reducing the risk of osteoporosis.

Exercise for Fat Loss

Exercise is an important component of any fat loss program, as it can help increase calorie burn and create a calorie deficit. Here are some types of exercise that can be effective for fat loss:

Aerobic activity: Any type of exercise that raises your heart rate and increases your breathing rate is aerobic exercise, also known as cardio. Examples include biking, swimming, running, and walking quickly. Cardiovascular health can be improved and calories burned through aerobic exercise.

High-intensity interval training (HIIT): HIIT involves alternating periods of high-intensity exercise with periods of lower-intensity exercise or rest. This type of exercise has been shown to be particularly effective for fat loss, as it can increase calorie burn both during and after the workout.

Resistance training: resistance training, also known as strength training, involves using weights or resistance to build muscle. Building muscle can increase your metabolic rate and help you burn more calories throughout the day.

Circuit training: circuit training involves performing a series of exercises with little to no rest between them.

This can help keep your heart rate up and increase calorie burn.

Walking: while it may not be as intense as some other types of exercise, walking can still be an effective way to burn calories and support fat loss. Make it your goal to walk for at least 30 minutes each day.

Make a workout buddy: Working out with a buddy can help you stay motivated and accountable. Consider finding a friend or family member who also wants to exercise and work out together.

Vary your workouts: doing the same workout every day can get boring and may also lead to a plateau in your results. Varying your workouts can help keep things interesting and challenge your body in new ways.

Incorporate activity into your day: in addition to formal exercise, try to incorporate more activity into your daily routine. This could include taking the stairs instead of the elevator, going for a walk during your lunch break, or doing some stretching while watching TV.

Remember, it's important to consult with a healthcare professional before starting any new exercise program, especially if you have any underlying health conditions or concerns. They can develop a safe and effective exercise plan that meets your needs and goals.

Fad diet and extreme measures

Fad diets and extreme measures for weight loss are approaches that are often popularized by the media, celebrities, or even some health professionals. These approaches may promise quick and significant weight loss, but they can also have negative effects on health and be unsustainable in the long term. Here are some examples of fad diets and extreme measures for weight loss:

Low-carb diets: low-carb diets restrict carbohydrates and can result in initial weight loss, but they may not be sustainable in the long term and can lead to nutrient deficiencies.

Detox or cleanse diets: these diets claim to "detoxify" the body and promote weight loss, but they often involve extreme calorie restriction, which can lead to nutrient deficiencies, dehydration, and loss of muscle mass.

Very low-calorie diets: these diets involve consuming fewer than 800 calories per day, which can lead to significant weight loss but can also lead to nutrient deficiencies, fatigue, and loss of muscle mass.

Liquid diets: liquid diets involve consuming only liquids such as shakes, soups, or juices, which can result in rapid weight loss, but they can also be deficient in essential nutrients and cannot be sustainable.

Extreme exercise: over-exercising can lead to injuries, burnout, and may not lead to significant weight loss if diet is not also addressed.

Surgery: Bariatric surgery is an extreme measure for weight loss that involves surgically altering the digestive system to restrict food intake or absorption. While it can be effective for significant weight loss, it carries risks and requires lifelong commitment to dietary and lifestyle changes.

Fad diets and extreme measures for weight loss can be tempting due to the promise of quick and significant results, but they often come with negative health consequences and may not be sustainable in the long term. A balanced diet and exercise plan, tailored to individual needs, is a safer and more sustainable approach to achieving and maintaining a healthy weight.

PART TWO: PRINCIPLES OF WEIGHT LOSS

CHAPTER FIVE

Setting Goals

Setting goals refers to the process of defining specific, measurable, achievable, relevant, and time-bound objectives that one wants to achieve within a particular timeframe. Goals can be short-term or long-term.

Setting goals is an essential part of personal and professional growth as it helps individuals to stay focused, motivated, and accountable. It allows you to have a clear vision of what you want to achieve, break down your aspirations into smaller steps, track progress, and celebrate successes.

Effective goal setting involves identifying SMART goals - goals that are specific, measurable, achievable, relevant, and time-bound. This means that goals should be clearly defined, quantifiable, realistic, aligned with one's values and priorities, and have a deadline for completion.

By setting goals, you can gain clarity, direction, and purpose, which can help you to improve performance, increase confidence, and achieve your desired outcomes.

Setting goals is an important step in achieving fat loss. Some tips for setting effective goals:

Be specific: set specific, measurable goals. Say, "I want to lose 5 pounds in the next few months."

Be realistic: set realistic goals that can be achieved with consistent effort. Avoid setting overly ambitious goals that may be difficult to achieve and may lead to frustration and disappointment.

Set short-term and long-term goals: set both short-term and long-term goals to stay motivated and track progress. Short-term goals can be achieved in a few weeks or months, while long-term goals may take several months or even a year to achieve.

Focus on behaviors, not just outcomes: instead of solely focusing on weight loss, focus on behaviors that can lead to weight loss. For example, aim to eat more vegetables, do strength training two times per week, or walk 10,000 steps per day.

Write down your goals: writing down your goals can help you stay accountable and track progress. Place your written goals somewhere visible as a daily reminder.

Adjust as needed: be flexible and adjust your goals as needed. Life happens, and it is important to be able to adapt your goals to changing circumstances.

Recognize progress: Celebrate your progress, regardless of how little it is.

Recognize the effort you have put in and the progress you have made, and use this as motivation to continue moving forward.

Identify your why: understanding your motivation for fat loss can help you set more meaningful goals. Think about why you want to lose weight or improve your body composition, and use this motivation to set specific and achievable goals.

Use the SMART criteria: when setting goals, use the SMART criteria to ensure they are Specific, Measurable, Attainable, Relevant, and Time-bound. This can help you set clear and achievable goals.

Break down larger goals: if you have a larger goal, such as losing 50 pounds, break it down into smaller, more manageable goals. For example, aim to lose 5-10 pounds per month, which can be achieved through a combination of diet and exercise.

Plan for obstacles: identify potential obstacles that may prevent you from achieving your goals, such as a busy work schedule or social events. Plan ahead to overcome these obstacles by scheduling workouts in advance or bringing healthy snacks to social gatherings.

Get support: enlist the support of friends, family, or a coach to help you stay on track with your goals. Having a support system can provide accountability and motivation to keep going.

Track progress: track your progress towards your goals using a food diary or fitness app. Seeing how far you've come can help you stay motivated to keep going.

By setting effective goals for fat loss, you can stay motivated, track progress, and achieve sustainable results. Focus on behaviors that can lead to weight loss, be flexible and adaptable, and celebrate your progress along the way.

Remember that setting goals for fat loss is a personal process, and it may take some trial and error to find what works best for you.

Important of Setting Goal

Setting goals is important for several reasons, particularly when it comes to achieving fat loss. Here are some key reasons why setting goals is crucial for success:

Motivation: goals can provide motivation and direction, giving you a clear idea of what you want to achieve and why. Having a goal can help you stay focused on the changes you need to make to achieve fat loss, and can help you stay motivated to continue making progress.

Accountability: setting goals can provide accountability, both to yourself and to others. By setting a goal and sharing it with others, you are more likely to stick to your plan and make the necessary changes to achieve fat loss.

Measurable progress: goals provide a way to measure progress towards achieving fat loss. By setting specific goals, you can track your progress and make adjustments to your plan as needed to continue making progress.

Improved confidence: achieving goals can help boost confidence and self-esteem. Seeing progress towards fat loss goals can help you feel more in control of your health and well-being, which can improve your overall quality of life.

Long-term success: setting goals can help you create healthy habits that can lead to long-term success. By setting specific goals and focusing on sustainable changes to your diet and exercise habits, you can achieve fat loss and maintain a healthy weight over time.

In summary, setting goals is an important part of achieving fat loss. Goals provide motivation, accountability, measurable progress, improved confidence, and long-term success. By setting specific, achievable goals and focusing on sustainable changes to your lifestyle, you can achieve your fat loss goals and improve your overall health and well-being.

Types of goal

There are different types of goals you can set when it comes to achieving fat loss. Here are some common types of goals to consider:

Outcome goals: outcome goals are focused on the end result you want to achieve, such as losing a certain amount of weight or fitting into a certain size of clothing. These goals are important for providing direction and motivation, but they can also be challenging to achieve because they are dependent on factors outside of your control, such as your body's normal response to exercise and diet.

Performance goals: performance goals are focused on improving your skills or abilities related to fat loss. For example, you might set a goal to run a 5K or to be able to do 10 push-ups. These goals are based on your own personal progress and are more within your control than outcome goals.

Process goals: process goals are focused on the actions you need to take to achieve fat loss. For example, you might set a goal to eat five servings of vegetables per day, to do strength training twice per week, or to walk 10,000 steps per day. These goals are important for creating healthy habits that can lead to sustainable fat loss over time.

Short-term goals: short-term goals are focused on achieving specific results within a shorter time frame, such as losing 5 pounds in a month. These goals can help you stay motivated and track progress, but they should be part of a larger, long-term plan.

Long-term goals: long-term goals are focused on achieving results over a longer period of time, such as losing 50 pounds in a year. These goals can provide direction and motivation, but they can also be challenging to achieve without breaking them down into smaller, more manageable goals.

When setting goals for fat loss, it's important to consider what type of goal will be most effective for you. Outcome goals can provide motivation, but it's important to focus on process and performance goals as well to create sustainable, healthy habits that lead to long-term success.

CHAPTER SIX

Food Quality vs Food Quantity

 Both food quality and food quantity are important factors to consider when it comes to weight loss. However, food quality plays a more critical role in achieving sustainable weight loss and overall health.

Food quality refers to the nutrient density and overall nutritional value of the food you consume, whereas food quantity refers to the amount of food you eat. Eating a diet that is high in nutrient-dense foods such as fruits, vegetables, lean proteins, and whole grains, can help you feel more satisfied, reduce cravings, and promote long-term weight loss. In contrast, consuming a diet that is high in processed foods, refined sugars, and unhealthy fats can lead to weight gain and other health problems.

While it's important to monitor your calorie intake to achieve weight loss, solely focusing on food quantity can lead to feeling deprived, which can increase the likelihood of binge eating and ultimately result in weight gain. Therefore, it is crucial to prioritize food quality over food quantity for sustainable weight loss.

Food quality is crucial for weight loss because it not only impacts the number of calories you consume but also affects how full you feel after eating. Nutrient-dense foods are generally high in fiber, protein, and other important nutrients that can help you feel satisfied and reduce hunger levels. In contrast, processed foods and high-sugar items can cause blood sugar levels to spike and then crash, leading to increased hunger and cravings.

Focusing on food quality can also help improve overall health and reduce the risk of chronic diseases such as heart disease, type 2 diabetes, and certain cancers. Consuming a diet that is high in whole, unprocessed foods can provide the body with the necessary nutrients for optimal health.

In terms of food quantity, it's important to keep in mind that everyone's caloric needs are different, and calorie counting is not always necessary or effective. Rather than focusing on the specific number of calories, try to eat mindfully, paying attention to hunger and fullness cues, and practicing portion control.

It's also important to note that the quality and quantity of your food are not the only factors that affect weight loss. Other factors that can impact weight loss include physical activity, sleep, stress levels, and hormonal imbalances.

Regular physical activity can help increase metabolism and burn calories, making it an important part of any weight loss plan. At least 150 minutes a week of moderate-intensity activity, such as brisk walking, cycling, or swimming, should be your goal.

Chronic stress can also impact weight loss by increasing levels of the hormone cortisol, which can promote fat storage and cravings for high-calorie foods. Finding healthy ways to manage stress, such as meditation or talking with a therapist, can help support weight loss efforts.

In summary, while food quality and quantity are important for weight loss, it's important to consider other factors that can impact weight loss success, such as physical activity, sleep, and stress management. By addressing these factors along with your diet, you can create a comprehensive weight loss plan that promotes long-term success and optimal health.

CHAPTER SEVEN

Creating Calories Deficit

Calorie deficit occurs when you consume lesser calories than your body needs to maintain its current weight. If you consume fewer calories than your body requires, your body will use the calories you have stored up to provide energy. You will lose weight as a result.

Creating a calorie deficit is a crucial component of achieving fat loss. Here are some strategies for creating a calorie deficit:

Track your calorie intake: start by tracking your current calorie intake for a few days to get a baseline of how much you're currently eating. There are many apps and websites available that make calorie tracking easy.

Reduce portion sizes: one simple way to create a calorie deficit is to reduce your portion sizes. Try using a smaller plate, or measuring your food to make sure you're not eating more than you need.

Choose lower calorie foods: opt for foods that are lower in calories, such as vegetables, fruits, lean proteins, and whole grains. Avoid high-calorie, processed foods that can be easy to overeat.

Increase your activity level: exercise can help create a calorie deficit by burning more calories. Walk for at least 1 to 3 hours of moderate-intensity exercise per week, such as brisk walking, cycling, skipping or swimming.

Increase your non-exercise activity: non-exercise activity, such as standing, walking, and fidgeting, can also help create a calorie deficit. Look for ways to be more active throughout the day, such as taking the stairs instead of the elevator, or taking short walks during breaks.

Use a food scale: using a food scale can help ensure you're accurately measuring your portions, which can help create a calorie deficit.

Plan your meals and snacks: planning your meals and snacks can help ensure you're making healthy choices and sticking to your calorie goals. It can also help prevent overeating and impulse eating.

Eat more protein: eating protein can help you feel full and satisfied, which can help you eat fewer calories overall. Aim for protein sources such as lean meats, poultry, fish, eggs, tofu, and legumes

Reduce your intake of high-calorie beverages: beverages can be a significant source of calories, especially sugary drinks like soda and fruit juice. Try replacing high-calorie beverages with water, unsweetened tea, or black coffee.

Be mindful of added sugar: added sugars can be found in many processed foods, and they can contribute a significant amount of calories to your diet. Read food labels and look for products with less added sugar.

Limit your intake of high-fat foods: high-fat foods, such as fried foods and fatty meats, can be high in calories. Try to limit your intake of these foods and focus on healthier fats, such as those found in nuts, seeds, and avocado.

Remember that creating a calorie deficit should be done in a healthy and sustainable way. It's important to fuel your body with nutritious foods and not drastically restrict your calorie intake, as this can lead to nutrient deficiencies and other negative health consequences. A gradual reduction in calories, coupled with regular exercise, can help you achieve fat loss in a safe and sustainable way.

Calories In vs. Calories Out

The concept of "calories in vs. calories out" is the basic principle of weight loss, which states that to lose weight, you need to consume fewer calories than you burn. This means that you need to create a calorie deficit by burning more calories through physical activity and exercise, while also consuming fewer calories through your diet.

However, it's important to note that the "calories in vs. calories out" concept is a simplified view of weight loss, and there are many other factors that can influence your body's ability to lose weight, including genetics, hormones, sleep, stress, and medications.

It's also important to focus on the quality of the calories you consume, rather than just the quantity. Eating a diet that is high in nutritious, whole foods can help support weight loss and overall health, while consuming a diet that is high in processed, high-calorie foods can make weight loss more difficult.

Overall, creating a calorie deficit by burning more calories than you consume is an important part of weight loss, but it's just one piece of the puzzle. A comprehensive approach that includes a healthy diet, regular exercise, and other healthy lifestyle habits can help you achieve your weight loss goals in a safe and sustainable way.

Calculating Calorie Needs

Calculating your calorie needs is an important step in creating a calorie deficit to support fat loss. There are several factors that can influence your calorie needs, including your age, gender, height, weight, and activity level.

One way to estimate your daily calorie needs is to use a calorie calculator, which takes these factors into account to give you an estimate of how many calories you need to maintain your current weight. From there, you can create a calorie deficit by consuming fewer calories than your maintenance level.

To use a calorie calculator, you will need to input your age, gender, height, weight, and activity level. Your activity level is based on how active you are during the day and can range from sedentary (little to no activity) to highly active (very active job and regular exercise). Once you input this information, the calculator will estimate how many calories you need to maintain your current weight.

It's important to remember that these calculations are just estimates and may not be completely accurate for everyone. Additionally, the level of calorie deficit you create will depend on your weight loss goals, as well as your ability to maintain a healthy and sustainable diet.

If you are unsure about how many calories you need to support your weight loss goals, it's a good idea to consult with a registered dietitian or healthcare professional. They can provide personalized recommendations based on your individual needs and help you create a plan that supports your overall health and wellbeing.

Strategies for Reducing Caloric Intake

Reducing caloric intake is an important part of creating a calorie deficit to support fat loss. Here are some strategies you can use to reduce your caloric intake:

Focus on whole, nutrient-dense foods: eating whole, unprocessed foods that are high in nutrients can help you feel full and satisfied with fewer calories. Whole grains, fruits, vegetables, lean proteins, and healthy fats are all good choices.

Practice portion control: pay attention to the amount of food you are eating and try to eat smaller portions. Use smaller plates and bowls, and measure out your food to avoid overeating.

Limit high-calorie, low-nutrient foods: foods that are high in calories but low in nutrients, such as sugary drinks, desserts, and fried foods, can add a lot of calories to your diet without providing much nutritional value. Try to limit your intake of these foods.

Eat slowly and mindfully: eating slowly and mindfully can help you enjoy your food more savory and become more aware of your hunger and fullness cues. This can help you avoid overeating and support healthy eating habits.

Drink plenty of water: drinking water can help you feel full and satisfied, and it can also help prevent dehydration, which can sometimes be mistaken for hunger.

Cook more meals at home: cooking your own meals can give you more control over the ingredients you use, and can help you avoid high-calorie restaurant meals.

Plan and prep your meals: planning and prepping your meals in advance can help you avoid making unhealthy food choices when you are short on time or feeling hungry.

Keep track of what you eat: keeping a food diary or using a food tracking app can help you become more aware of what you are eating and make it easier to identify areas where you may be consuming too many calories.

Limit alcohol intake: alcoholic drinks can be high in calories and can also lower your inhibitions, making it more difficult to make healthy food choices.

Be mindful of condiments and sauces: condiments and sauces can add a lot of extra calories to your meals. Be mindful of how much you are using and look for lower-calorie options.

Be aware of hidden sources of calories: some foods, such as granola, trail mix, and smoothies, can be high in calories even though they are marketed as healthy options. Be aware of the calorie content of the foods you are consuming.

Choose low-calorie snacks: snacks can be a major source of extra calories in your diet. Choose snacks that are low in calories and high in nutrients, such as fruits, vegetables, and low-fat yogurt.

Be aware of emotional eating: emotional eating can lead to consuming extra calories when you are not actually hungry. Be aware of your emotional triggers and find other ways to cope with your emotions, such as exercise or meditation.

Remember, the key to reducing caloric intake is to make small, sustainable changes to your diet that you can stick with over the long-term. Over time, even minor adjustments can lead to significant outcomes.

PART THREE : CONCLUSION

CHAPTER EIGHT

Building a Sustainable Lifestyle

When it comes to losing weight and keeping it off, it's important to focus on building a sustainable lifestyle that supports healthy habits for the long-term. Here are a few tips for building a sustainable lifestyle:

Focus on progress, not perfection: losing weight and building healthy habits can take time, and it's important to be patient with yourself. Rather than striving for perfection, focus on making progress and celebrating small victories along the way.

Find a workout you enjoy: exercise is an important part of a healthy lifestyle, but it's also important to find a form of exercise that you enjoy. This can help make it easier to stick with your routine over the long-term.

Plan your meals: planning your meals in advance can help you make healthier choices and avoid impulsive decisions. Take some time each week to plan out your meals and snacks, and consider prepping meals in advance to make healthy eating easier.

Get support: building a healthy lifestyle can be challenging, and it can be helpful to get support from friends, family, or a support group. Consider joining a weight loss or fitness community, or working with a healthcare professional or registered dietitian to develop a personalized plan and get support along the way.

Set realistic goals: setting realistic, achievable goals can help you stay motivated and make progress towards your weight loss and health goals. Rather than setting unrealistic goals, focus on small, achievable changes that you can sustain over the long-term.

Practice self-care: practicing self-care, such as getting enough sleep, managing stress, and engaging in relaxing activities, can help support healthy habits and improve overall well-being.

Stay hydrated: drinking enough water is important for overall health and can also help support weight loss efforts. Aim to drink at least 8 cups of water a day, and consider incorporating low-calorie beverages like unsweetened tea or flavored water to mix things up.

Practice mindful eating: mindful eating is the practice of paying attention to the present moment and being aware of the food you're eating to avoid overeating. Try to eat without distractions, savor your food, and pay attention to hunger and fullness cues.

Be flexible: a sustainable lifestyle is one that allows for some flexibility and occasional indulgences. Rather than restricting yourself completely, aim for a balanced approach that allows for some treats and indulgences in moderation.

Make it a habit: building healthy habits is key to maintaining a sustainable lifestyle. Make healthy eating and regular exercise a habit by incorporating them into your daily routine, and find ways to make it enjoyable and sustainable for the long-term.

Individualization: fat loss strategies should be individualized to meet your unique needs, preferences, and lifestyle. There is no one-size-fits-all approach to fat loss, so it is important to find what works best for you.

Remember, building a sustainable lifestyle is a process, and it's important to be patient with yourself and focus on progress, not perfection. By making small, sustainable changes and focusing on building healthy habits over time, it's possible to achieve long-term weight loss and improved health.

Lifestyle Changes for Fat Loss

Lifestyle changes are key to achieving and maintaining fat loss over the long-term. Here are some lifestyle changes that can support fat loss:

Increase physical activity: regular physical activity is essential for fat loss and overall health. Aim for at least 150 minutes of moderate-intensity exercise per week, or 75 minutes of vigorous-intensity exercise per week, as recommended by the World Health Organization.

Eat a healthy, balanced diet: eating a healthy, balanced diet is important for achieving and maintaining fat loss. Focus on whole, nutrient-dense foods, including fruits, vegetables, lean protein, whole grains, and healthy fats. Avoid highly processed foods and foods high in added sugars and saturated fats.

Get enough sleep: lack of sleep can disrupt hormones that regulate appetite, leading to increased hunger and overeating. Aim for 7-9 hours of sleep per night to support fat loss and overall health.

Prioritize self-care: self-care is important for overall health and can support fat loss efforts. Take time to engage in activities that you enjoy, such as reading, spending time outdoors, or spending time with loved ones.

Keep a food journal: keeping a food journal can help you become more aware of what you're eating and make healthier choices. Write down what you eat and drink each day, along with the time of day and any notes about how you're feeling. This can help you make adjustments.

Practice portion control: portions control is important for managing calorie intake and supporting fat loss. Use smaller plates and bowls, measure out servings, and avoid eating straight from the package to help control portion sizes.

Incorporate strength training: strength training is important for building lean muscle mass, which can help increase metabolism and support fat loss. Aim to strength train at least 2-3 times per week, focusing on exercises that target all major muscle groups.

Reduce screen time: spending too much time in front of screens can contribute to a sedentary lifestyle and increase the risk of weight gain. Limit your screen time and find other ways to be active, such as going for a walk, playing with your kids, or gardening.

Remember, lifestyle changes take time and effort, but they can lead to sustainable fat loss and improved health over the long-term. Start by making small, achievable changes and focus on progress, not perfection. By building healthy habits and making lifestyle changes that support fat loss, you can achieve your weight loss goals and improve your overall well-being.

Building Habits for Success

Building healthy habits is an essential part of achieving and maintaining fat loss. Here are some strategies for building habits that can support your weight loss goals:

Start small: begin with small, achievable goals and build from there. For example, aim to drink more water or take a 10-minute walk each day. Small changes can add up over time and lead to lasting results.

Make it a routine: incorporate healthy habits into your daily routine to make them easier to stick to. For example, plan your meals and snacks ahead of time, or schedule your workouts at the same time each day.

Use positive reinforcement: reward yourself for sticking to your healthy habits. This could be something small, like a relaxing bath or a favorite TV show, or something larger, like a massage or new workout gear.

Get support: enlist the help of friends, family members, or a coach to support you in your weight loss journey. Having someone to talk to and hold you accountable can help keep you motivated and on track.

Track your progress: keep track of your progress to see how far you've come and stay motivated. This could include taking measurements, weighing yourself, or tracking your workouts and meals in a journal.

Plan for setbacks: setbacks are a normal part of any journey, so plan for them in advance. Create a plan for how you'll get back on track if you slip up or face a challenge.

Focus on consistency, not perfection: remember that progress is more important than perfection. Don't let small setbacks derail your efforts, and focus on consistently making healthy choices over time.

Prioritize sleep: getting enough sleep is crucial for weight loss and overall health. Aim for 7-9 hours of sleep each night, and create a relaxing bedtime routine.

Practice stress management: stress can lead to overeating and weight gain, find healthy ways to manage stress. This could include exercise, meditation, deep breathing, or spending time with loved ones.

Choose whole, nutrient-dense foods: focus on eating whole, nutrient-dense foods that support your health and weight loss goals. This includes foods like fruits, vegetables, whole grains, lean protein, and healthy fats.

Stay hydrated: drinking plenty of water can help you stay full, reduce cravings, and support weight loss. Aim for at least 8-10 glasses of water each day, and consider adding in other hydrating drinks like herbal tea or sparkling water.

Find movement you enjoy: exercise doesn't have to feel like a chore. Find movement you enjoy, whether that's dancing, hiking, or weightlifting, and make it a regular part of your routine.

Practice self-care: taking care of yourself can help you feel more confident and motivated on your weight loss journey. This could include things like taking a bubble bath, getting a massage, or treating yourself to a healthy meal.

Seek professional help if needed: if you're struggling to make progress on your own, consider seeking professional help. This could include working with a registered dietitian, personal trainer, or therapist to help you reach your goals.

Overcoming Obstacles

Making lifestyle changes and working towards fat loss can be challenging, and it's normal to face obstacles along the way. Here are some tips for overcoming common obstacles:

Lack of motivation: if you're feeling unmotivated, try setting small goals and celebrating your progress along the way. You can also find an accountability partner, such as a friend or family member, to help keep you on track.

Cravings: to manage cravings, try incorporating more filling, nutrient-dense foods into your diet. You can also try distraction techniques, such as going for a walk or calling a friend, to help take your mind off of food.

Time constraints: if you're struggling to find time for exercise or meal prep, try breaking your routine down into smaller, more manageable chunks. You can also consider outsourcing tasks, such as hiring a meal delivery service or a cleaning service, to free up more time.

Plateaus: if you're not seeing progress, try mixing up your routine by trying a new type of exercise or experimenting with different foods. You can also reevaluate your goals and make sure they're realistic and attainable.

Negative self-talk: it's important to be kind to yourself and avoid negative self-talk. Focus on your progress and celebrate your successes, no matter how little.

Social pressure: sometimes social situations, such as going out to eat with friends or attending parties, can make it difficult to stick to your fat loss goals. In these situations, try to plan ahead and make healthy choices whenever possible. You can also communicate your goals with your friends and family and ask for their support.

Stress: stress can make it harder to stick to healthy habits. To manage stress, try incorporating relaxation techniques, such as yoga or meditation, into your routine. You can also prioritize self-care, such as getting enough sleep and taking time to do things you enjoy.

Lack of knowledge: if you're not sure where to start, consider working with a personal trainer or registered dietitian. They can provide guidance and support to help you reach your goals.

Lack of support: having support from friends and family can make a big difference when working towards fat loss. If you're not getting the support you need, consider joining a support group or online community where you can connect with others who are working towards similar goals.

Injuries or health issues: if you have an injury or health issue that makes it difficult to exercise or follow a certain diet, talk to your healthcare provider. They can provide guidance on how to stay active and healthy while working with your individual needs and limitations.

Overcoming Setbacks and Challenges

Overcoming setbacks and challenges is an important part of any fat loss journey. For overcoming obstacles, consider these suggestions:

Identify the setback: the first step in overcoming a setback is to identify what caused it. Was it a lack of motivation, an injury, or a change in your routine? Once you know what caused the setback, you can work to address it.

Reframe your mindset: instead of viewing setbacks as failures, try to reframe your mindset and view them as opportunities to learn and grow. Use setbacks as a chance to reflect on what went wrong and what you can do differently moving forward.

Adjust your plan: if you've experienced a setback, it may be necessary to adjust your plan. This could mean modifying your exercise routine, changing your diet, or adjusting your goals. The key is to be adaptable and willing to make adjustments as necessary.

Be patient: fat loss is a journey, and setbacks are a natural part of that journey. Remember that progress takes time, and be patient with yourself as you work to overcome challenges and reach your goals.

Celebrate your successes: even small successes can help you stay motivated and on track. Celebrate your accomplishments along the way, whether it's reaching a new milestone in your fitness routine or making healthy food choices.

CHAPTER NINE

Encouragement and Next Step

Congratulations on starting your weight loss journey! It takes a lot of effort and dedication to commit to a healthier lifestyle. Here are some words of encouragement and next steps for your weight loss journey:

Be patient and consistent: remember that weight loss is a journey, and it takes time to see results. Don't get discouraged if you don't see progress immediately, and keep up with your healthy habits.

Set achievable goals: setting small, achievable goals will help you stay motivated and focused. Don't be too hard on yourself if you make a mistake; instead, celebrate your progress.

Focus on healthy habits: rather than just focusing on losing weight, focus on building healthy habits that will support your overall health and well-being. Get enough sleep, exercise frequently, and eat a healthy diet.

Find a support system: having a support system can help you stay accountable and motivated. This could be a group of people you know, family, or even online.

Consider working with a professional: a registered dietitian or a personal trainer can provide guidance and support as you work towards your weight loss goals.

Get active: exercise is an important component of weight loss and can help you burn calories and build muscle. Have a target of at least 15 - 30 minutes of moderate activity daily.

Limit processed foods: processed foods are often high in calories, sugar, and unhealthy fats, so try to limit your intake of these foods and focus on whole, nutrient-dense foods instead.

Stay motivated: find sources of motivation that work for you, such as setting a specific goal, rewarding yourself for progress, or finding a workout buddy.

Developing Long-Term Habits: one significant disadvantage of dieting is the lack of a plan for transitioning off the meal plan. Most eating plans include what to eat while following them, but what you eat afterward is just as important. This is why it is preferable to choose an eating plan that you can stick to for the rest of your life.

Don't Stop Exercising: if you used exercise to help you achieve your weight loss goals, stopping abruptly without making changes to your eating plan may result in weight gain. This occurs because fat loss requires more calories burned than consumed. If you are burning fewer calories but still exercising, weight gain may still occur.

To keep your weight stable, you must consume the same number of calories as you burn during the day. You should avoid making drastic changes to your diet and exercise routine. Instead, make gradual changes that will not result in significant weight gain. Allow yourself 6–8 weeks to reach your maintenance level.

It might be easier for you to lose weight than to keep it off. Weight maintenance takes a lot of time and effort. That is why it is critical to devise a strategy to help you maintain your weight loss and achieve your health objectives.

Take Note of What You Eat: don't rebound and revert to your old eating habits after losing weight.

Take an 80/20 approach: a sustainable meal plan includes foods that you enjoy. It is a combination of nutritious foods that keep you full and satisfied, as well as some comfort foods. The 80/20 rule states that 80% of your meals should be balanced and nutritious, while the remaining 20% should be less healthy foods.

This could mean eating balanced meals throughout the week and having pizza night with your family on Fridays, or having a drink or two with your buddies on the weekends. The key is to cultivate the mindset that all foods have a place in a well-balanced diet.

Be ready for setbacks: it is normal to experience setbacks such as a plateau or weight fluctuations. It's how you handle setbacks that makes all the difference.

Find healthy alternatives to your favorite foods: instead of cutting out your favorite foods altogether, try finding healthier alternatives. For example, you can make homemade versions of your favorite takeout meals using healthy ingredients.

Instead of giving up in frustration, keep your cool and continue on your path. Any changes in body weight usually disappear within three to five days. If the scale continues to rise above that point, it could indicate muscle gain or increased body mass.

Non-scale victories, such as how good you feel in your clothes or having the energy to chase after your children, can serve as reminders of your progress. Give yourself some grace if you find yourself feeling guilty about overindulging. Reminding yourself that a setback is not the end of the world, try relieving stress and don't give up.

Remember that weight loss is a journey, and it's important to be patient, consistent, and kind to yourself. Focus on making sustainable lifestyle changes that will support your overall health and well-being and don't be afraid to ask for support when you need it. With dedication and hard work, you can achieve your weight loss goals!

www.ingramcontent.com/pod-product-compliance
Lightning Source LLC
Chambersburg PA
CBHW050825250726

48653CB00006B/2437